I0435804

What's It *Really* Like?
Pregnancy & Birth

M.D. BOWDEN

What's It *Really* Like? Pregnancy & Birth

Published by M.D. Bowden

Copyright © M.D. Bowden 2013

All rights reserved

M.D. Bowden has asserted her moral rights to be
identified as author of this work.
No part of this work may be reproduced without prior
permission in writing from the author.

ISBN-13: 978-1491084540

ISBN-10: 1491084545

BY M.D. BOWDEN

The Two Vampires:
Dark Wine
Dark Blood
Dark Love
Dark Moors

First in New Series – Out Now!
Gateway to Faerie

Non-fiction:
What's It *Really* Like? Pregnancy & Birth

Table of Contents

What's It *Really* Like?
Pregnancy & Birth

For Daisy

Chapter 1: School Days

I had always wanted a baby. When I was eleven years old I fantasized about becoming pregnant. Being incredibly naive, much like Winona Rider's character in the film Mermaids, I wondered of highly impossible ways I may have conceived following my first kiss. I imagined it would be bliss having a baby inside me. Heavenly. Nothing could be more amazing than nurturing a life – holding a hugely swollen belly and feeling it move as a tiny baby kicked inside.

I grew up in a small rural town in Devon, England. It is called Hartland. There was a shop called 'Pop-in', a chippy called 'Shamrock café' and a post office. Oh, and three pubs.

I went to the local primary and knew the local kids. I lived with my mum and younger sister in a new four bed on the edge of town. My parents had divorced when I was eight, and me and my sister visited our father at weekends.

The house we lived in with our mother backed onto fields – I used to watch the cows lining up to be fed from my bedroom window. Just around the corner was the entrance to the woods - a beautiful expanse of oaks with a stream meandering through the centre, 'The Vale', as it was known locally. I've no idea if that's its real name.

I loved walking in the woods, and when I was at primary school I loved playing in them. My sister, my best friend and I used to make camps. Thinking back on it; I'm amazed we had so much freedom. We didn't make camps with our parents, no; we went into the woods for hours on our own, building stream side dens and camouflaging them with leaf litter so we wouldn't be noticed. It was great fun.

It was in those same woods that I used to imagine walking with my baby – the baby I longed for and frequently dreamt of. I would walk through these woods, in my mind, holding a beautiful baby in a sling – tightly against my chest.

It was a tranquil vision. It was freedom – with love and compassion thrown in.

Did I think of how heavy it would be carrying a baby through the woods? No! Did I imagine that baby crying, constantly trying to sooth it - my stress levels ready to go through the roof? No!

Did I imagine how hard pregnancy would be? The morning sickness that would last for nine – no – *ten* months? After all – pregnancies last 40–41 weeks. Did I imagine the heartburn, or the thighs so large they chaffed as I walked? No!

My point is – nothing was remotely like I ever imagined, and that is why I am writing this story. It is a true story – an honest account of pregnancy and birth. My intention in revealing my experiences is not to scare would be mothers, it's to educate - so they know what to expect. That way it's possible to be mentally prepared.

I will try and cover the main points I wanted to know when I was pregnant – not the science, which is easy to find out, and not the week by week accounts you can read in any pregnancy magazine – the gritty stuff! Sure – it's different for everyone. Some people may have absolutely delightful pregnancies, along with pain free births, but I'm sure that's not the norm!

**

I didn't get pregnant when I was eleven.

I finished primary school and went to the local secondary. Now – this was not your usual school. Most kids from Hartland were bused to comprehensives in Bideford or Bude, but my sis and I went to 'The Small School', which was only a five minute walk away. To get there I walked down one long street, past two of the three pubs, plus the two shops I mentioned.

The school was in an old converted chapel and had a grand total of forty students. My class was the biggest – there were ten in my year. It was indeed much like a family as everyone knew everyone. The school day started with 'circle', where the head teacher played the guitar and sang folk songs, while we all pretended to join in. This was followed by a talk by one of the other teachers. I seem to remember most of the talks being about travels in India, where two of our teachers had previously lived, and where the founder of the school had been a Jain monk. This cultural education was followed by a minute of silence.

Yes, it was most definitely a hippy school. We only had lessons in the morning, students cooked vegetarian meals everyone had to eat – packed lunches were not allowed. The meal was preceded by a prayer that ended in 'peace, peace, peace'. In the afternoon we did sewing, or yoga, or pottery – then had to join our allocated teams to clean the school. I remember plenty of dust.

Someone I met while at this school had quite an impact. She was a teacher at the time - not one of our main teachers, but someone who came in to help out on occasion. She was from Hawaii – I thought her beautiful, and her husband was a very attractive artist. They had three kids and I thought they were the perfect family. One day when I was visiting their house she showed me a portrait of herself when she was pregnant. In the picture she was fully naked, standing half way up their stairs at an angle to the camera – the pose accentuating her beautiful bump. I've always remembered that photo and the longing it brought – how much it made me want to be pregnant. See – I didn't just want a baby – I actually longed to be pregnant.

So I got through school and went to college, but I didn't meet any suitable men to have a baby with! Of course – I did think of other things too – I didn't really think I was going to have a baby when I was that young, however tempted I was. I also wanted a career, although I changed my mind every five minutes about what I thought that career might be, being fixated on finding the perfect one.

***

It wasn't long after college when I did meet someone. He was a musician in a band my friends were crazy about.

He was the one, and I fell hopelessly in love – but there was a slight hitch – he had a girlfriend! So I went about my life with an aching heart, trying to find my path in life – not knowing what to do at all. Me and this man remained close friends, regardless of the fact he had now moved to London where he was studying music at Westminster University. I still saw him in the holidays – often enough that I couldn't forget about him in order to fall for anyone else in a serious way.

It was some five years later, when I was living in a little chalet on a holiday park with my two cats, and planning on attending university myself that September, that he came to stay and we finally got together. Yay! And years later together we still are – we have two children and are just engaged – I know, wrong order and all . . .

So my man moved in, but there was that slight hitch that I was about to start University. I didn't want to give up on that idea. I won't say dream – it was a practical choice. I was going to study dietetics, but not for any inspired reason – I was interested in nutrition and I thought being a dietician would be a career I could handle – and I needed to do something!

He agreed to come with me, so off we went to Plymouth in South Devon. We rented a flat and he got a job. I started University. His first job was awful – having a degree in music wasn't proving very useful. He worked behind the bar in a club where if a lady were to, let's say – stand on a table and take off her top – she would be awarded a bottle of bubbly. He had to stay there until four in the morning. It wasn't great. His next job was at a farm shop working as a butchery assistant. This was better, he didn't actually mind the work itself, and we got to eat lots of tasty organic meat – but he often had to work six long days a week and he was utterly bored of it. He applied for other jobs more related to his interests but to no prevail.

I was doing OK at Plymouth Uni. I'd made friends and was getting good marks, but it was awfully dull. Plus – I didn't learn anything about nutrition. I was very disappointed by the course content, and – I probably shouldn't say – but the teaching didn't do it for me. I stuck the first year, passed all the exams – I just had the placement to get through. This was a hospital placement in the summer holidays, and I had to go to Poole hospital on the South coast. What a shock I got! Being a dietician was a completely different job to that which I had thought it was. Going into it I thought the job of a dietician was to sit in an office and see patients – who you would question and give advice. It turns out this is only part of the job of being a dietician, and most of it requires working the wards, at least for the first few years. This was not what I had planned for myself – and not what I wanted at all. I trailed around on my placement, talking to patients – watching the elderly being given energy supplements they usually refused to drink, and trying not to throw up as we went to see people in the gastric ward. I'm not very good at dealing with the sound of constant retching.

I didn't quit there and then. I went back to University and started my second year. The content was a little more interesting, although we still didn't learn much about nutrition - we learned about diseases and talking to people. Plus there were some science classes, biochemistry – that kind of thing – relatively interesting, but not really helpful for actually being a dietician. Each time I came home from University I was fuming about the course and the fact I thought we were really learning the wrong stuff. It was all so basic and patronising!

I guess it was about this time that my man suggested we try for a baby. He actually suggested it – not me!! Oh my God – I had a man asking me if I wanted to have a kid with him. Years of longing for a baby, and was I going to say no? No! Of course not.

Regardless of the fact I was angry at the course I was doing, I was still determined to continue as I'd already given up on other career ideas, and I didn't know what else to do. I thought I would get pregnant and continue doing the course. Well, I actually thought it would take a long, possibly very long, time to get pregnant. This was partly why we decided to go for it. You see – we had a couple of friends who had been trying for a baby for years and not succeeding, and they started trying when they were about thirty. We didn't want to wait until we were older and risk not having kids.

We decided to start trying for a baby straight away, so I stopped taking the progesterone only pill I was on. Two weeks later . . .

Chapter 2: Pregnancy

I started to get cramps, and feel a sinking depression. It hadn't worked – I wasn't pregnant – I was going to get my period. I forced myself out of bed regardless, and suffered the thirty minute walk to University. I had a practical class that morning of a dietetic nature – we had to weigh ourselves and measure various body parts. The idea was that if we practiced on each other we'd be more adept when it came to using the weird prong things on patient's bellies, backs and arms - to measure their body fat content.

I sat down next to a friend and duly complained about period pains. She offered me some Ibuprofen which I took thankfully. We teamed up and were given a list of all the fatty areas we had to measure. Every girl's dream ;)

This was the second time we had had that practical. The last time was the previous week, so we already had a list of measurements to compare. We went for the bog standard scales and I weighed myself first as my friend was more embarrassed about her weight than I was. She was perfectly thin, but the week before we had discovered that my BMI, or Body Mass Index, was lower. When I'd weighed myself that week I had been about ten stone. I'm nearly six foot tall.

When I stepped on the scales I thought - that's odd. I was ten and a half stone.

I'd put on half a stone.

Oh well, these things happen, I thought. Maybe it was water retention of something.

On to the next machine – the body fat analyser. We read the instructions and it said 'do not use if you think you may be pregnant'.

'Well, that's not me,' I thought, and stepped on. As I was standing on the machine, thinking that my boobs felt kinda tender and wishing that the ibuprofen would kick in, and the fat analyser was doing its job, a dawning thought occurred to me – Shit – what if I am pregnant? I quickly brushed that thought aside, thinking it couldn't be true, and remained standing on the machine.

My fat content had increased. Hmmm.

We went around all the other areas, wrestling with the tape measures and prongs. A growing battle was raging in my mind. Could I be pregnant? No – don't be ridiculous – it's too soon. By the end of the class I was quick to leave, and dashed to Boots to buy a pregnancy test.

I had to know for sure.

An hour later and I was at home peeing on a stick. This is harder than it sounds – you've got to be quite accurate as you have to pee directly on a small area of the stick for at least five seconds. It's pretty hard not to pee on your hand. As someone who's now done their fair share of pregnancy tests, I fully recommend peeing into a clean jar and sticking the test in there. It's far less messy.

I placed the freshly peed on test on the edge of the sink, and did my best not to stare at it for the minute it took to work - the minute that felt like an eternity.

When the time was up I looked at the stick. It was one of the ones that had two boxes – one had a line on it to say that the test had worked, the other would have a line in it if you were pregnant, or no line if you weren't. It was supposed to be clear cut – the line would either be there or it wouldn't.

I looked at the test very closely, holding it in the light by the window. Was that very faint pink mark a line? No, I decided – it wasn't, I wasn't pregnant. I went and had a cup of tea, then went back to the test and studied it again.

The mark looked a little bit more like a line.

Hmmm, was I imagining it? Was it just wishful thinking? Could I be pregnant?

There was one thing for it – I would have to get more tests!

I went back to Boots and bought five tests. One of which was more expensive but said it would be able to tell if you were pregnant up to one week before your period was due.

I rushed home and did three tests. They were all positive.

Oh my God, I was pregnant.

I was buzzing with excitement and disbelief – we'd been trying for two weeks! Shit.

I called my partner and shakily told him. He couldn't believe it either – and said I should do more tests. I reassured him I had already done four, and they said they were ninety-nine per cent accurate.

This was the point worry started kicking in. What about the fact I went on the fat analyser machine, when it said not to if you were pregnant? Would my baby be OK? Why was I hurting so much? My womb area still felt mightily uncomfortable – surely that wasn't normal? I started looking on-line for information about pregnancy symptoms to find out what *was* normal. That was when I read you're not supposed to take Ibuprofen when pregnant – as it increases the chance of miscarriage. What if the pain I was having was because I was losing the baby?

I rang the doctor.

I got an appointment that day and trundled off down to the University surgery where the doctor told me, 'Yes, you are pregnant.' That comment wasn't courtesy of an examination, or anything like that, but was based on the fact I'd done a home test. He said he'd transfer me to a midwife, and that he didn't know if I was losing the baby – I would have to wait and see.

On that positive note I went home and curled up on the sofa in pain. I summed up the courage to ring my mother, who used to be a GP and had now turned homoeopath. She actually wasn't that surprised I was pregnant, and was reassuring about my pain. She looked on-line herself and found cases where bad cramps were also experienced, and everything turned out fine.

***

Me and my man had recently bought a house and were in the middle of renovating it, so it was quite a mess. That was just before the bank crisis, when they'd give anyone a mortgage, and we took out a large one. So I walked through the dust of our project and crawled under the covers. The pain got worse and I didn't manage to go to University for a few days. I lay in bed crying in pain, and wracked with worry.

After a few days it started to ease, and I hadn't had any bleeding so began to feel more positive. But then I started to feel sick, not really badly, but it was pretty much constant. The smell of paint and varnish really made me feel bad. I tried to go to a lecture at Uni but had to run out halfway through as I felt like I was going to vomit.

I made an appointment with my tutor to explain the situation. We met up in a café near the University where I forced myself to sit, fighting nausea. She was very understanding and we agreed that I would take some time off, and I would come back when I started to feel better.

I didn't start to feel better, I felt really crap and pretty depressed about being stuck at home.

The weeks past and me and my partner talked about what we should do. Should we stay in Plymouth? Did I really want to finish my degree? Did it seem likely I would manage to finish it anyway – now that I was pregnant? Wouldn't I want to stay home and look after our baby?

If I left University, and my NHS grant stopped, would we even be able to pay our mortgage? We realised we wouldn't be able to, and we were in a bit of a pickle.

Then a job opportunity came up as a Music Technician at The Plough Arts Centre in Torrington, Devon, in the same town my mother now lived in. My man applied and he got the job. That settled things, I left the University and we moved back to the chalet, which was in commuting distance of his new job. We rented out our house.

***

It was nice being back in the chalet, and forgetting the pressures of Plymouth. Our view was beautiful – it looked out across the ocean, with woodlands on either side. There were gorgeous walks within a hundred metres. Sure, it was a little small, and the bathroom was off the living room, but it felt like home.

In the years before I had started Plymouth University I had been studying for a degree at The Open University. I had already completed my first two years, so decided to resume my studies. It would give me something to while away the hours while I was waiting to have the baby, but it would involve taking an exam six weeks after the birth. I decided to go for it, as I felt like needed to work towards something.

Regardless of doing this the weeks went by so slowly. I read everything I could about the birth and pregnancy, and a little about looking after babies. This was so abstract though, and was hard to take in without any immediate practical application.

After the first twelve weeks of pregnancy the nausea did begin to improve. I found that if I ate regularly, and picked on things like crystallised ginger, it helped. Salty crisps were good too. I tried to eat healthily and walked as much as possible. I felt tired most of the time, but I wasn't working, so I could rest after exercise.

At about twelve weeks I had my first scan.

I was incredibly nervous – what if there was something wrong? What if the Ibuprofen, the fat analyser, the alcohol – all the things I may have done wrong before I knew I was pregnant – had had some adverse effect on our baby?

We had to go to the hospital for the scan, and it was combined with various tests like blood pressure and urine. The wait was excruciating. It was at least two hours before we went in. This isn't good when you're pregnant, feeling sick, faint, and nervous. But it was worth it when we saw the tiny heart beating on the screen – our baby was OK. My blood pressure was very low – too low. That was probably one of the reasons for the dizziness.

Soon I was in the second trimester, which was definitely the best part of being pregnant. I felt slightly less sick, my tummy was starting to round out and the baby inside me had started to kick. It was very strange when this first happened – it felt like little bubbles popping in my lower abdomen. It did feel amazing that there was a life inside me.

I started to have weird dreams. I remember one when I dreamt I gave birth to a fish! I guess I still couldn't quite believe I was really having a baby. Right the way through the pregnancy I felt that way, and I was constantly waiting for something to go wrong.

At about twenty weeks into the pregnancy we had the second scan – the one where we could find out the sex of the baby. I was really excited and nervous. I was still worried they would find something wrong as they would be looking at the baby and taking measurements, checking for Down's syndrome or spinal bifida I think. We talked about whether we should find out the sex of the baby before-hand, but it wasn't really a big dilemma. We decided it would be a surprise whenever we found out, and if we knew sooner we would get a chance to prepare.

I really wanted a girl, and I really didn't want a boy! I was worried I wouldn't know how to relate to a boy baby, and I guess I still had the childish fantasy of dressing my girl in pretty clothes and playing with her hair.

When we saw the baby on the screen it was amazing – not only could we see and hear the heart beating, but we could see the hands, feet and head. The scanner couldn't see a penis, so thought the baby probably was a girl, but we couldn't be sure. We got photos to take home and show our family.

***

It was around this time that clothes started to be an issue. I couldn't get away with any of my jeans anymore, and it was hard to find any decent maternity clothes in Barnstaple – which was the closest large town. In the end I discovered the best thing was to wear loose dresses with leggings.

When my mother was pregnant she got really bad varicose veins, and she got stretch marks too. I wasn't as bothered about the idea of stretch marks, as I'm not really a bikini gal, although I did want to do my best not to get them. Every day I would massage cocoa butter stretch mark cream into my tummy, or natural lotions from Lush, to help prevent myself from getting them.

I *really* didn't want to get varicose veins. Any chance I got I would elevate my legs above my waist, and I would never stand still for long. Even in the shower I would constantly move and stretch my legs.

Whether it was from these measures I took, or whether I was just lucky, I don't know – but I didn't get varicose veins or stretch marks at all. Phew.

Showers also made me very dizzy, I couldn't stay in for long or I would literally have to get down on my hands and knees to stop myself from fainting. I tried various things, like eating before I got in the shower to make sure my blood sugar levels weren't too low, but nothing worked. Baths had the same effect, but we didn't have one in the chalet anyway.

***

Going into the third trimester I was starting to get really big, my hip was beginning to twinge and I felt pretty gassy. Not nice. These things just got worse as the trimester progressed. I'd put on more weight than recommended, as I was still nibbling constantly to fight nausea. I was also very hungry – would wake up in the night starving and I would have to eat, so I had a stash of bananas and cereal bars by my bed. This is completely not normal for me, I had never had to eat in the night before.

The worst thing that kicked in around this time was the heartburn. It started mildly in the second trimester, but got worse into the third. As the baby gets bigger it starts pressing up against your diagram and stomach – restricting this area. I felt short of breath, and with the gassiness and heartburn my chest often felt tight. I was frequently worried I was having a heart attack. I'd have to lie down to try and relax my chest or I'd often start to feel really sick. But I couldn't lie down! The heart burn was so bad I'd need to prop myself up in bed with lots of pillows, even at night. This made it very hard to sleep. My overactive mind didn't help the situation – I was constantly thinking about childbirth, wondering what it would be like and wondering what it would be like looking after a baby. I bought Gaviscon to deal with the heart burn, and had to take frequent gulps. This did help, but it tasted disgusting and generally made me feel more bloated and sick. I had milk by my bed, to try before resorting to Gaviscon. The milk sometimes did the trick.

I had the book 'What to Expect When You're Expecting'. It was quite information packed, but a slightly depressing read. I thought it focused more on the problems that might occur, and it had the tendency to make me feel more paranoid. I read about the birth a lot and bought endless baby magazines. I read lots of stories about people having incredibly quick births and not even making it to the hospital. I wondered if we should have a home birth as I didn't relish the idea of the forty minute drive to Barnstaple hospital while in labour. I also read plenty of stories about women who had had pain free births. This filled me with hope. Apparently – if I got into the right state of mind – if I was relaxed enough, kept the lights low and didn't have too many interventions, it was possible birth could be pain free.

I spent a lot of time researching all the things we needed for having a baby, and the things I would need to pack for the birth, in case we did need to go to the hospital. I had the hospital bag packed from about thirty weeks in – in case the baby was early.

I was constantly expecting to go into labour. I was having 'Braxton Hicks' contractions, which weren't really painful - more like gentle tightening's of my abdomen – not as painful as I'd remembered Rachel's were in the American TV show 'Friends'. But as I was hoping for a pain free birth I kept thinking - what if they were real contractions - how was I supposed to tell?

My mother reassured me I *would* be able to tell, but could I trust her? Wasn't every labour different? How would I really know?

I didn't want to go overboard with the things I bought for the baby, worried that if I bought too many things it would jinx it, how bad would I feel if I had a chalet full of baby equipment and no baby? But there were certain things I would need. We got a moses basket and baby blankets. Lots of baby grows and nappies. Maternity pads for the post birth bleeding that would occur and breast pads for mild leakages.

I had read that some people start to produce milk early – before the baby was even born. I kept looking at my nipples to see if I was starting to make milk. I also had read about the possibility of perineal tearing during birth. It had happened to my Mum. It filled me with dread. She had informed me that having her tear sewn up was more painful than the birth. But then – she had had an epidural as her blood pressure had been high. As the end of my pregnancy neared I rubbed olive oil into my perineal area, the bit of skin between the vagina and anus, to try and prevent tearing.

My baby was kicking lots – it was quite painful sometimes – especially when I was kicked in the ribs. But I was pleased when I felt kicking as it reassured me the baby was OK. However when it kicked lots I worried something was wrong, as I'd read when the baby is in distress it might kick more than usual!

I spent a lot of time just holding my tummy, thinking about the baby that was inside, talking to it, stroking it – trying to bond before the birth. I would play classical music to try and stimulate its mind and increase its intelligence.

My tummy was getting really big and it was becoming hard to walk anywhere. My hip pain was really increasing – it was OK when I was still, but when I walked it was really painful. Apparently this pain is caused by the hormone relaxin as it prepares your body for the birth – loosening the joints so the baby will have room to get out.

My thighs were so large that when I walked they rubbed against each other uncomfortably. My man took me for very slow walks to try and keep me in some form of shape. After all - I had read that the better shape you were in, the easier the birth would be. However this was becoming very challenging – I knew I was far from in good shape.

I started to feel really sick in the evenings. It kicked in around dinner time, and every two to three days I would feel so bad I would actually be sick. It was mainly retching, and gassiness, but it was horrible. I hate being sick. After I was sick I tended to feel improved, but I felt drained and miserable – when was this going to end?

***

We planned for a natural birth. Of course – it was going to be pain free – but if it wasn't I would be fine, I would be able to handle it. I would not get an epidural. I would not take drugs. I didn't want to do anything that could have an adverse effect on the baby. I didn't want to risk intervention as I had read it would increase the risk of having a caesarean, and I was intent my baby would come into this world in the most natural and peaceful way possible.

I was equipped with soothing music and homoeopathic remedies – I would be OK.

Chapter 3: The birth

My due date came and went. I read about all the ways to stimulate the birth; from sex, to walking, to curry. We tried them all, but nothing worked. Then my mum gave me a homoeopathic remedy that was supposed to induce birth. I was a week overdue at that point, and if I hadn't gone into labour I was going to have to see the midwife the following day for a 'sweep'. That involves the midwife sticking her hand up your vagina and doing something to the membranes. Fortunately I didn't get to have this pleasure, as whether through the effects of my mothers remedy, or because the natural time had come – I had the first sign of labour.

It was five 'o' clock in the morning on the following day. I woke up needing to pee, as was pretty constant during the whole pregnancy, and went into the bathroom. There was a smear of blood in my pants – something I had read was called a 'show' and meant that the birth was imminent.

I went back to bed and woke my partner. He asked if I was having contractions, I said no, he rolled over and went back to sleep. Charming.

I lay in bed, propped up on all those pillows, unable to go back to sleep. I was waiting for something to happen – what would it be first – would my waters break? Would I get contractions? Shit, what if I was already having contractions but they were so pain free that I couldn't feel them, what if I was already ten centimetres dilated and I was about to pop out a baby?

At nine 'o' clock I woke up my partner. Those were the days. Lie-ins . . .

I insisted he call the midwife. I wasn't having contractions yet, but he should tell her I had had a 'show' and ask if we still had to come in.

She said we didn't, so we stayed at home waiting for something to happen. We went for a walk, I ate a light breakfast as apparently it's good to eat to keep up your energy, but not good to eat too much as when all your blood rushes to your tummy during labour you may just be sick.

At about ten 'o' clock I started to feel mild abdominal pains – it was soon pretty clear that they were contractions. My partner rang the midwife and she asked to talk to me. Phone reception was an issue – it was very intermittent at the chalet. We had to go for a walk to use the phone, and I eventually talked to the midwife. I think she wanted to talk to me personally so she could gage how much pain I was in, and work out how soon a midwife visit would be required.

At this stage we were still planning on a home birth, although my hospital bag was ready – as it had been for the last eleven weeks. Along with all the baby paraphernalia, I had stuffed it with snacks like crisps, nuts and jelly babies – things that I could dig into to preserve my birthing energy. I'd put in some bottles of Evian and even some coke, as I'd heard the hospital water tasted disgusting.

The midwife decided she would visit to check on my progress – but not for two hours. Two hours! This filled me with panic – what if I was already labouring by then?

We were told that, even if we wanted to go to the hospital, it was too early on. We needed to time the contractions and not go anywhere until they were only five minutes apart.

We went back home and put on that relaxing music. I sat on a birthing ball and bounced a little. The pain got worse.

The pain got a lot worse.

By the time the midwife did turn up a few hours later my contractions were five minutes apart. It felt like my bladder was going to explode. Literally. I was really worried about it. Every time I had a contraction my man would hold onto my hand tightly and I would lean forward, holding my belly with my other hand and breathing through the pain.

Surely this was it. My contractions were every five minutes. I was in a lot of pain. I must be at least eight centimetres dilated. I *must* be ready to pop.

***

The midwife arrived at about three p.m. She saw my pain and decided an examination was in order. I lay back on my bed and took off my lower garments. She stuck her whole hand inside me. It didn't exactly hurt, but it was mightily uncomfortable.

After feeling around for a bit she extracted her hand and informed me I was one centimetre dilated. Yes, that's right. 1cm.

What? How was this possible? To be ready to give birth you have to be ten centimetres dilated.

'This is entirely normal,' she reassured me.

Then she informed me she'd be off – she'd come back in a few hours to see how we were doing. As we were still planning on a home birth, when she returned she would decide if it was time to call in another midwife. You have to have two midwives present for a homebirth.

The hours passed. The bladder that felt like it was going to explode continued to increase in pain. It was unbelievable. Unbearable. I needed an epidural. I couldn't handle it any longer. We rang the hospital and told them we were coming in.

My man went and put the hospital bag in the car. We had already put in a little car seat for our baby, so we would be able to bring it back from the hospital. Every time he left my side, even for a minute, panic rose inside me – what if I needed to push?

He came back for me and escorted me slowly to the car. I felt very self-conscious outside in so much pain. I had a contraction as we got to the car, and leant over – clutching on to the car door in agony. All my partner could do was hold on and rub my back, it was reassuring but certainly not adequate. Each contraction felt like an escalating pain that went on for ever. I think they only lasted a minute, which sounds completely bearable. Surely if it's only one minute of pain, every few minutes, you'll be able to handle it – right? That's what I'd thought anyway. I had just had no idea how intense the pain could be. A few years before

I had broken my ankle – the pain had been incredibly intense for a very short time. If I could liken the pain of birth to anything it would be to that, but that happening over and over again for hours and hours on end.

When that contraction eased I sat in the back of the car on a towel. I wanted to sit in the back as I thought I'd be less noticeable. It was about six p.m. and rush hour would just be dying down, so hopefully the traffic wouldn't be too bad.

All the stories I'd read about labouring women not making it to the hospital in time flashed through my mind. I really hoped we'd make it.

My man started the car and drove towards the hospital.

With each contraction I screamed out for him, clutching my belly and clawing at the seat back in front of me. How could the pain be so bad? Surely there was something wrong. I wanted to get to the hospital as fast as possible, then I would be there when my bladder actually did explode. I seriously thought this was a possibility.

My waters broke while in the car. It was a good job I'd been prepared and sat on that towel. They didn't burst in a gigantic splat, as tends to happen on television - I just started to leak liquid. Quite a lot of it, but it maintained its flow. I kind of felt like I was weeing myself, but I knew I wasn't.

The journey was as bad as I had feared. We had to pull up at traffic lights as we came into Barnstaple. We had people in front and behind as we waited for the lights to change. I had a contraction there and then – trying not to scream too loudly.

Finally we were at the hospital. It was evening so we could park near the maternity entrance rather than having to park in the car park. As I got out of the car I had another contraction, and again leant over the car crying in pain. As it eased we went into reception. Thankfully it was deserted as there were no evening appointments. It was the same place we had had to wait for the scans. We were ushered through to the maternity ward by a receptionist. You have to go through two sets of doors – presumably to block out the screams of labouring women from the pregnant mothers waiting for their appointments. I had another contraction before we even made it through the second door.

We got into the maternity reception and had to answer questions. They had to see how much pain I was in before deciding whether I was allowed a room. After another contraction someone promptly led us through to a room, informed us a midwife would be in to see us soon, and left us alone. I was boiling hot. I was so hot. I striped off all my clothes. I didn't care anymore.

'I need an epidural,' I cried to the midwife as she entered.

'We'll see,' she said. 'Let's examine you first.'

Another hand inside me.

'You're two centimetres dilated. It's too early for an epidural – try some gas and air,' she said.

They don't like you to have an epidural too early on as it can slow the birth and lead to complications – like a caesarean.

She showed us how to use the gas and air and told us she'd come and check on us later.

As the next contraction hit I sucked on the gas and air machine. It made me feel sick. It didn't help the pain. I tried again for a few more contractions but it was no good, I was in so much pain – I really needed an epidural. The midwife came in and saw me mid contraction. I was leaning on the bed screaming in pain. She tried to tell me to calm down, that it was early on and I needed to get a grip. OK, so those probably weren't her actual words – but I felt like they were. The midwife wasn't one of those motherly figures – she was more like Professor McGonagall from Harry Potter. Nice and well meaning, but strict and not very loving or reassuring.

She decided she would examine me again – as I insisted I must be close, it was so ridiculous to think that I wasn't.

She stuck her hand inside me again as I whimpered between contractions. I was five centimetres dilated. She looked slightly shocked as it wasn't long since she'd last examined me. She agreed to go and talk to the anaesthetist. She left us on our own.

Every time we were left on our own I thought I was going to have the baby. When she didn't return my man had to go and find her. I was entirely on my own then and I cried as the next contraction hit, trying to breathe through it, trying to cope, but let's be honest – I was a mess.

My man came back with the midwife and she informed me the anaesthetist was busy. Busy? No! This couldn't be true. When was he going to be free? 'Oh, in a few hours maybe.' What?

I had another contraction. I screamed. I cried. The midwife said I could have pethidine, which is a morphiate. Exactly what I didn't want after reading it could slow the babies breathing.

'Yes, give it to me,' I said, before screaming in pain again.

I really got the impression the midwife thought I was being pathetic, like I should be coping far better. She didn't seem to think my bladder would explode, and brushed this query aside.

She left the room and reappeared with a large needle. OK, so my memories may be a little hazy from here on –

but I remember the needle as being very large. A lot larger than a vaccination needle. I think she injected it into my thigh. I started to feel the effects immediately, and managed to sit on the edge of the bed. The pain didn't go away, but I became more detached from it, and I got very sleepy. My man continued to rub my back hard during contractions, and he held my hand between them. At some point he put on the relaxing music we'd brought. I promptly told him to turn it off.

After some extended period of blurry memories the pain started to get worse again.

'Epidural?' I asked again.

The midwife went to check.

The anaesthetist was still busy.

I was given more pethidine.

At some point the midwife returned and insisted I lay back on the bed. I didn't want to do this. I was still sitting on the side, refusing to move. I remembered, through my drug induced haze, that I had to give birth upright, or kneeling, or something. I couldn't lie down. That wasn't active birthing. I would be more likely to rip if I lay down.

'Yes, she told me – but you can't give birth sitting down either – how will the baby come out? And I need to examine you again,' she said.

During all this heart rate monitors were sporadically attached to my tummy to measure the babies heart rate, to make sure everything was OK. This is only a hazy memory though, it wasn't a big deal, and I was reassured to know that my baby was doing fine when I heard its heart beating.

My partner and the midwife made me move. They put me on my back on the bed, and she stuck her hand in me again. I was eight centimetres dilated. I was close.

Someone came in and said I could have an epidural. The midwife said it was too late, that I couldn't have one this close to delivering. That it would be dangerous to stick a needle in my spine when the contractions were so close together.

Some point not long after this I felt the urge to push.

'Don't push now,' I was told, 'you're not dilated enough.'

However - when the urge to push kicks in there's really not much you can do to stop yourself. It's pretty impossible not to push at all. It feels like your body is trying to make you do a really big poo and there's nothing you can do about it. I pushed as gently as I could. Fluids and blood and all sorts of ichiness flowed out of me. The midwife kept changing the hospital pads that were under me.

'You can get into an active birthing position now,' the midwife said.

I refused to move.

Eventually she said I could push. I pushed so hard, I pushed for my life, for the life of my baby. I felt good to push, incredibly, incredibly painful, but good. Like I was doing something, like this was it, and it was going to end. I was soon going to have a baby.

My partner was down the end with the midwife, watching between my legs as the baby crowned. Stinging pain engulfed me. I pushed as hard as I could. This was seriously the hardest thing I have ever done in my life. I pushed with all my might, like the world would end if I didn't.

The head came out and I cried. I had to wait in that position with the babies head, and the midwifes hands, between my legs until the next contraction came. I pushed again and out slid the rest of the baby. She was promptly placed on my naked chest, still attached to the umbilical cord. I cried, I can't remember if she cried. I hadn't checked but I knew it was a girl. She was covered in blood and I held her in an unbelieving shocked state. I tried to get her to attach to my boob, and the midwife helped. You are supposed to do this straight away as it will be calming for the baby, they get the nutrients they need from the colostrum, and it helps cause contractions in the uterus that will expel the after-birth.

There was so much blood, and pads were changed again. The umbilical cord was still attached as we'd read it was more natural to leave it for a bit.

Our baby was wrapped in blankets and my partner held her. He was so happy he cried. She was so small.

I thought I should ask – 'Is she a girl?'

'Yes, she is a girl.'

I tried to feed her again, which worked a little. The afterbirth still didn't appear though, and I was too tired. The midwife came with an injection. My man cut the cord and a white gauze plaster was placed over our babies belly button. He held her while the midwife injected me again, this time in my bum, I think.

I had to push again for the placenta to come out - it wasn't as hard as for the baby though. It came out, plus more blood. There was blood everywhere.

I was given back my girl and I held her, she was so squashed and purple and peaceful.

'I'm going to be sick!' I said, thrusting her into my partners arms, and promptly was.

I lay back on the bed, completely exhausted.

The midwife did the checks that were necessary for the baby. She was weighed and my man was helped by the midwife to dress her in a baby grow, with a little hat. He placed her in a little cot that was next to my bed.

I wasn't going to let her out of my sight – what if they got her confused with another baby?

I was given toast with honey, which I nibbled on – trying to feel better.

Our baby fell asleep in her cot.

She was amazing, so beautiful, I couldn't believe she was real. She was mine.

I think it was about two in the morning. The midwife said she would leave us alone to get cleaned up. Were we OK to go home? It would be possible to go up to the ward, although she made it clear this would be quite an inconvenience, and told us either way that we had to leave the room we were in, soon. We said we would go home.

I stumbled painfully into the adjoining bathroom and tried to wash off all the blood. My partner went out to the car to bring in the baby car seat, and then he started packing up our stuff. I felt abandoned and exposed, barely able to stand as I tried to get myself clean. It hurt so much in my nether regions. I tried to pee but it was unbearably painful.

When I had washed off all the blood I quickly put on some pants with a large maternity pad to catch the blood that was still leaving my womb. I dressed and joined my man, who was being helped by the midwife to strap in our little one into her car seat.

We left the hospital at four 'o' clock in the morning and returned to our chalet with our tiny baby sleeping in the back. I sat next to her and constantly monitored her breathing, staring at her face. Her little shiny button nose, her tiny fingers that were slightly blue and wrinkly. She clenched her fingers around my thumb. I was in love.

Chapter 4: Photos

♥

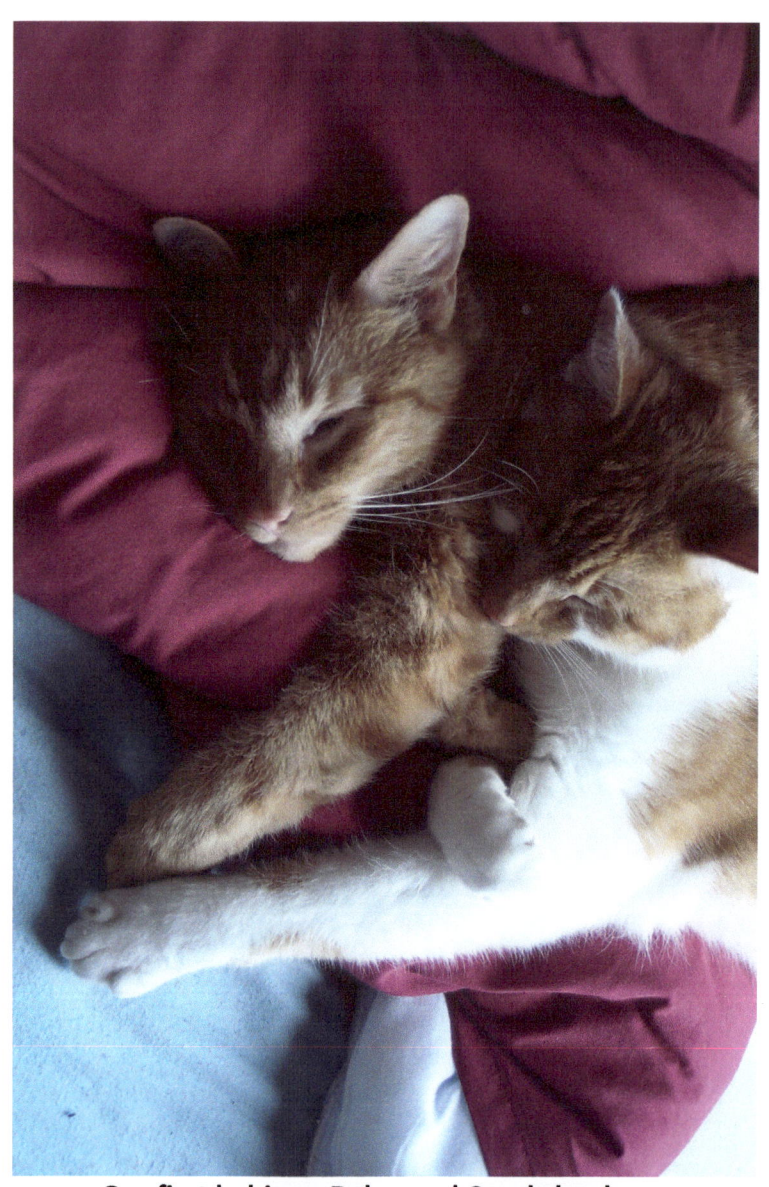

Our first babies – Dylan and Crookshanks

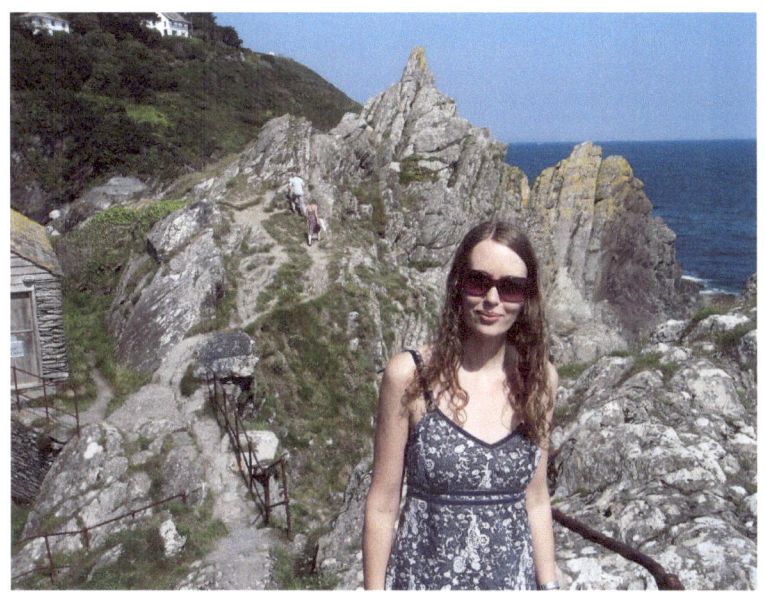

Me, shortly before I was pregnant

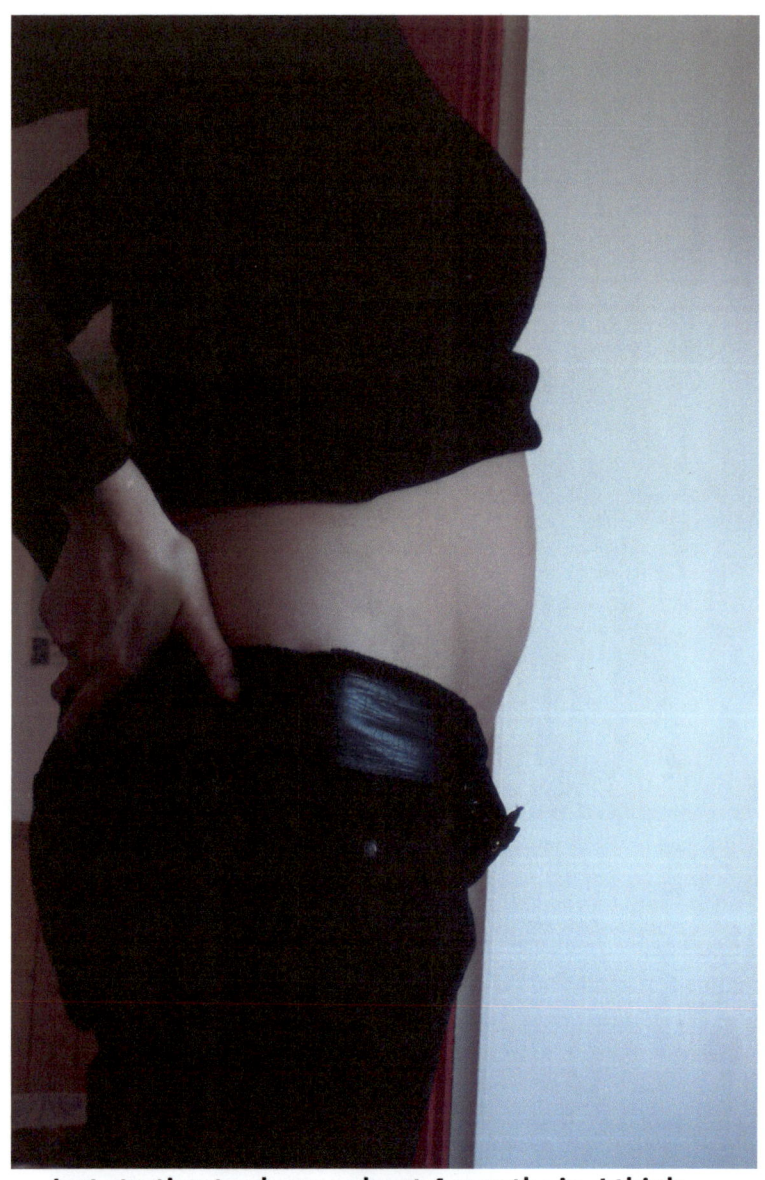

Just starting to show – about 4 months in, I think

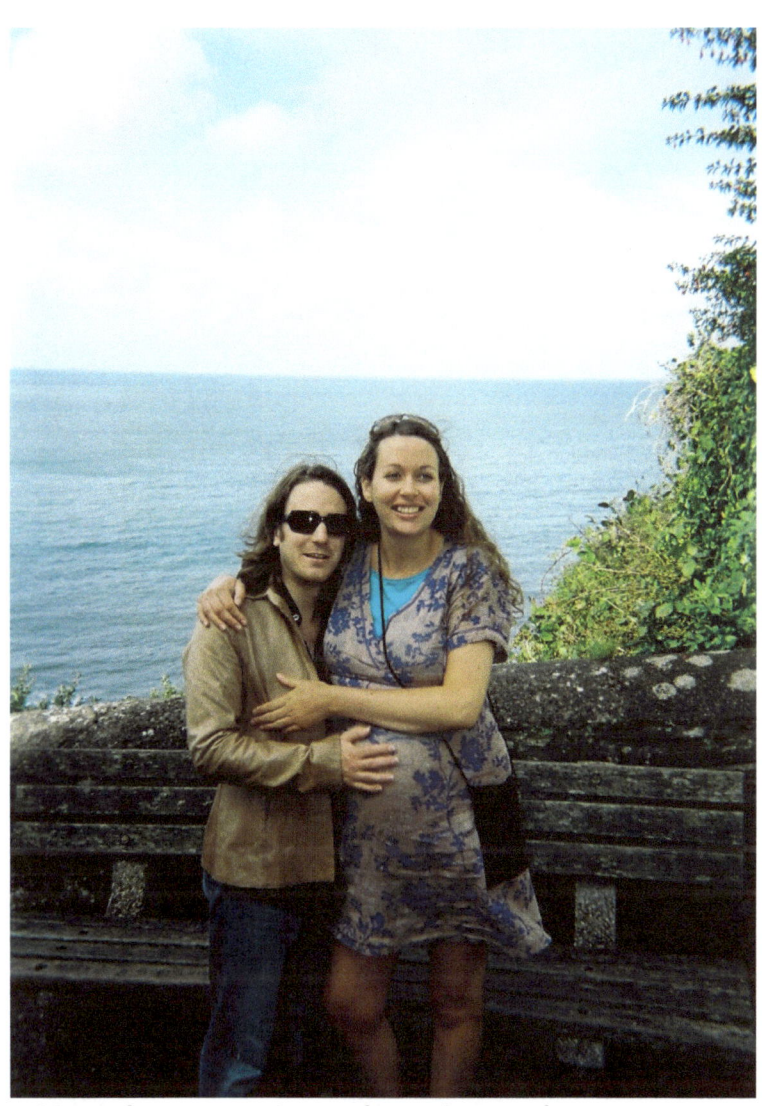

Me and my man – I was about six months pregnant

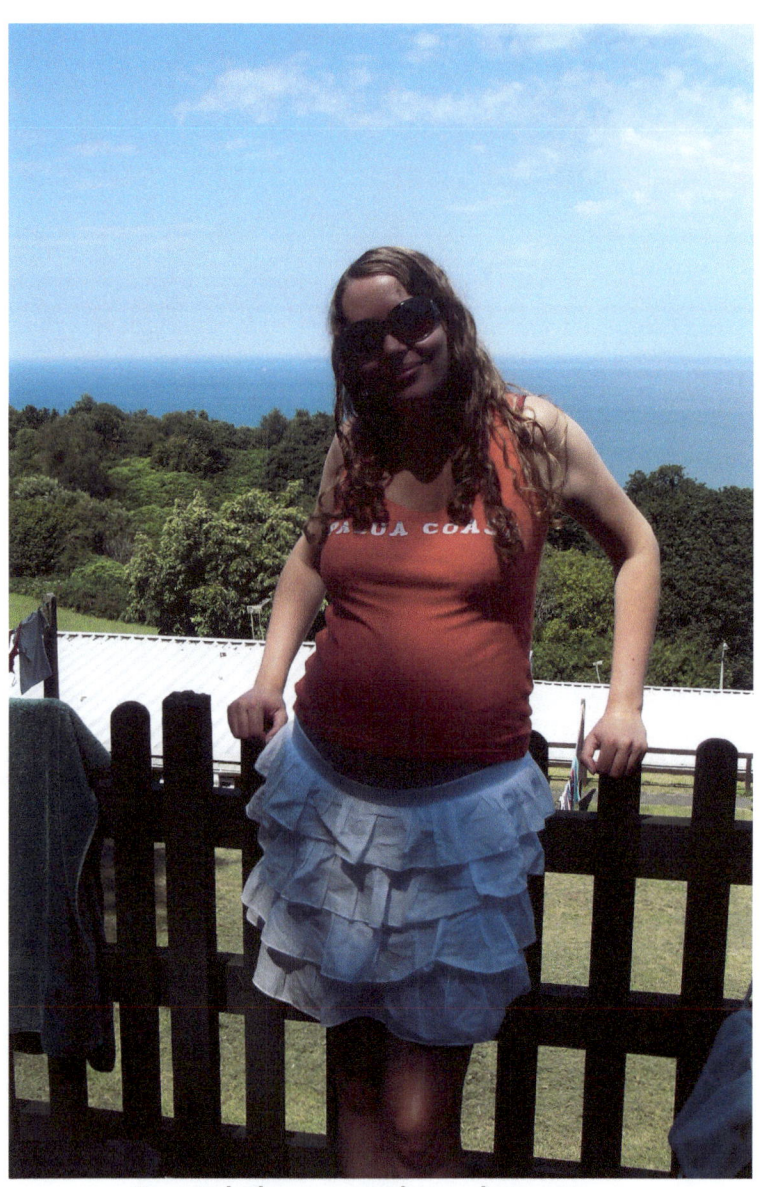

On our balcony, nearly ready to pop

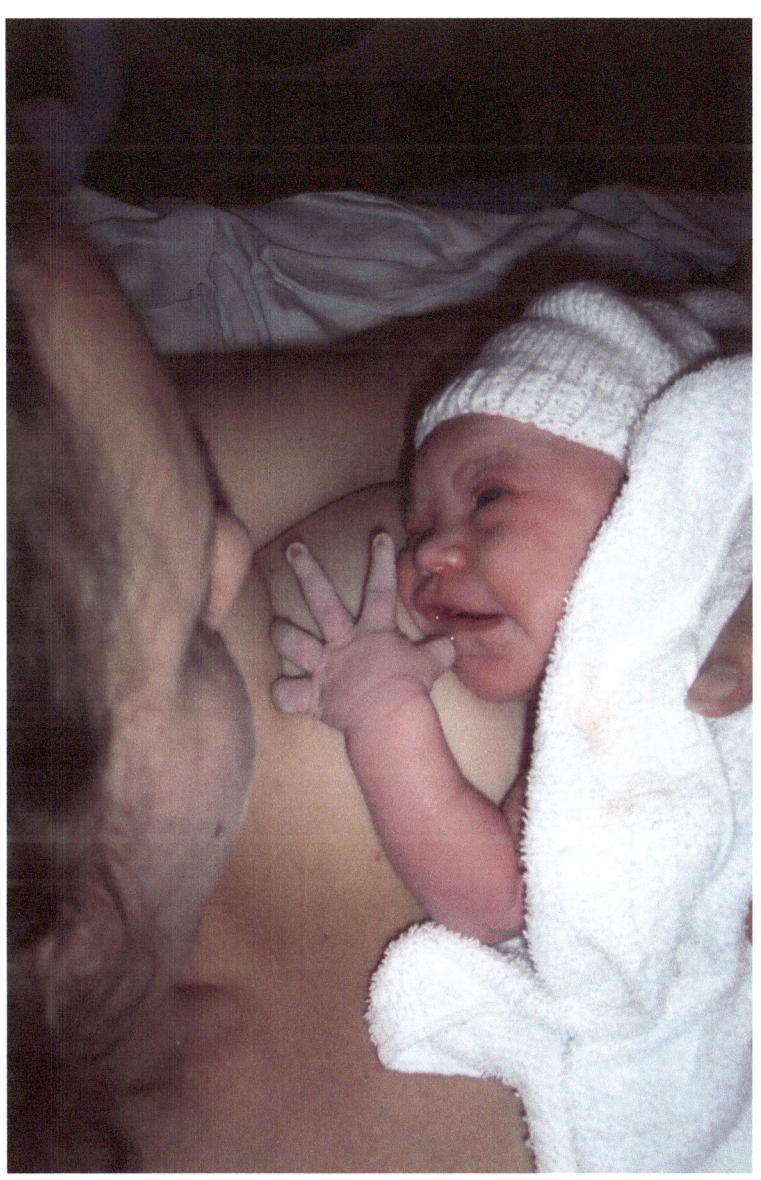

Me with our little one, just after she'd emerged

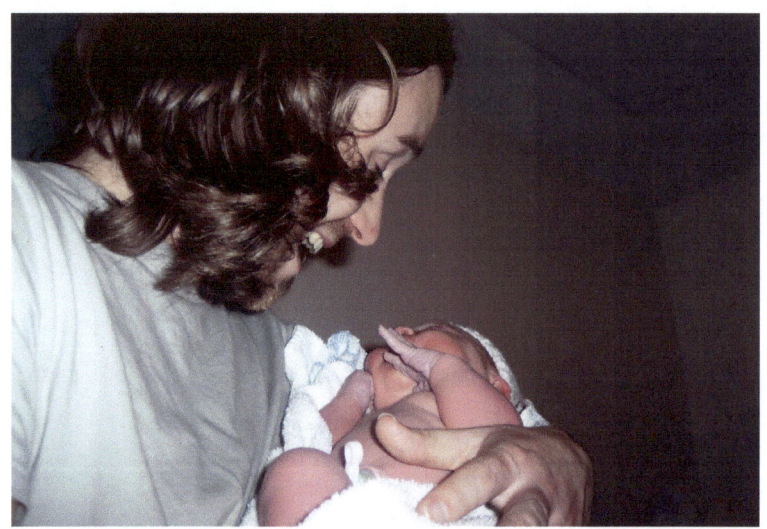

My man with our bubs

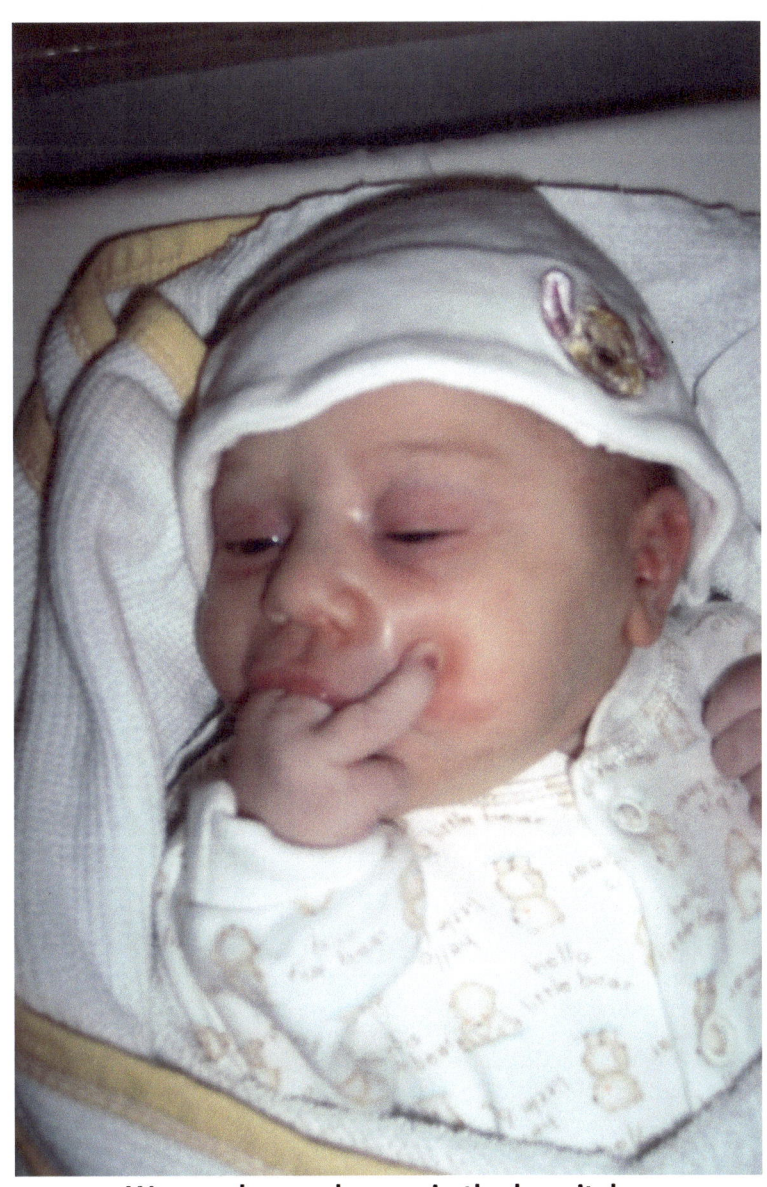

Wrapped up and warm in the hospital

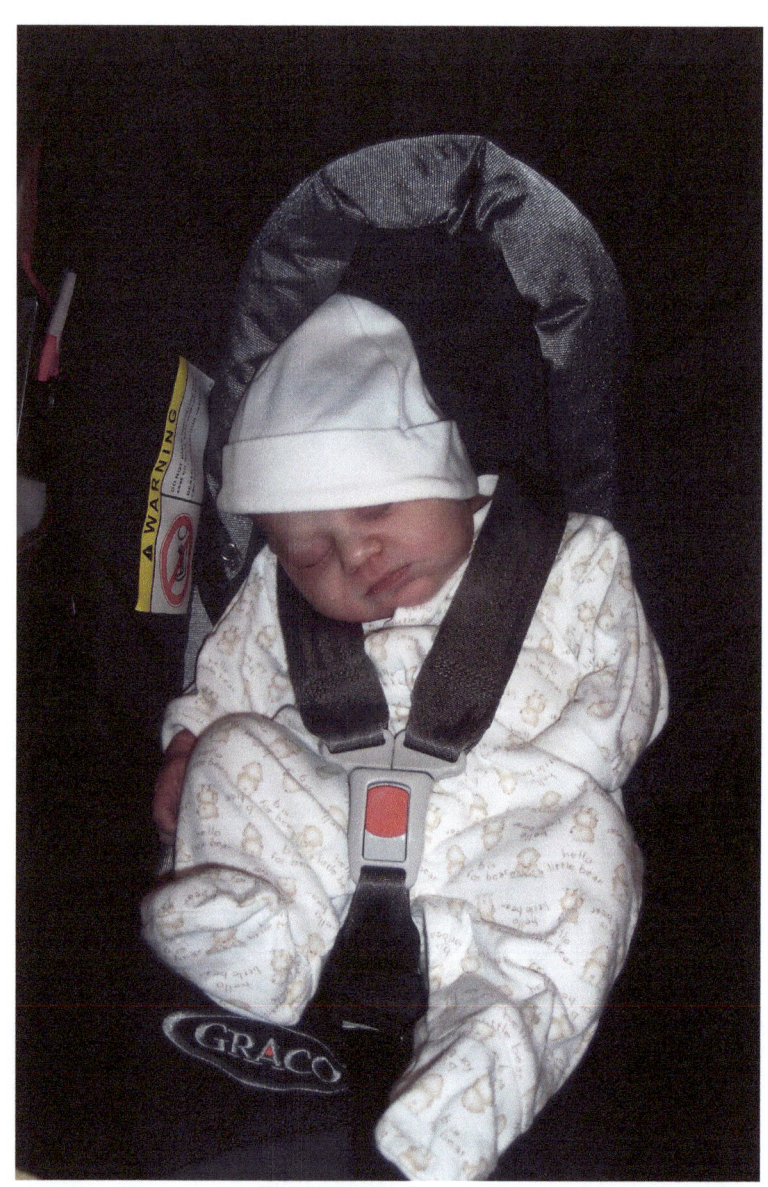

On our way home

Epilogue: 5 years later

Inow have two children; a girl and a boy. I breastfed my little girl until she was a year and four months old. When she was about nine months old, we decided to try for another baby! Two months later I was pregnant again. Pregnancy was pretty similar the second time around (except I was extra hungry because I was still breast feeding my daughter!), with the same ills and joys, but this time I was going to be more prepared for the birth. I was determined! I took up pregnancy yoga, and every day from about six months in, I listened to a hypnosis for birth cd. We had home birth. My partner, my mum and a midwife accompanied me, and delivered the baby. My partners' parents looked after my daughter during the process so she wouldn't be upset by the screaming. We warned the neighbours!

The whole thing was much easier the second time around. I had the hypnosis cd on repeat from the first contraction, right up until the baby was out. My little boy. I know second births are supposed to be easier anyway, but respective of this, I would definitely recommend anyone who is pregnant giving hypnosis a go. It didn't take away the pain, but it made it easier to cope with it mentally.

My daughter is now nearly five years old, and she is just about to complete her first year at school! My son is three years old, and a very cheeky boy! One day I may write a book about the home birth, and looking after babies and young children, but for now this is the end of my story. If you are pregnant, and near to giving birth yourself, I wish you the best of luck – and I hope my truthful account hasn't scared you too much! I hope knowing how painful birth can be helps prepare your mind for birth, and helps prevent you being as horrified and scared as I was the first time around. Just remember – it's completely normal for it to be unimaginably painful! It doesn't mean that anything is wrong. Most of all, I hope you have a good birth experience and enjoy being a mum!

THE END

For other books by M.D. BOWDEN keep on turning . . .

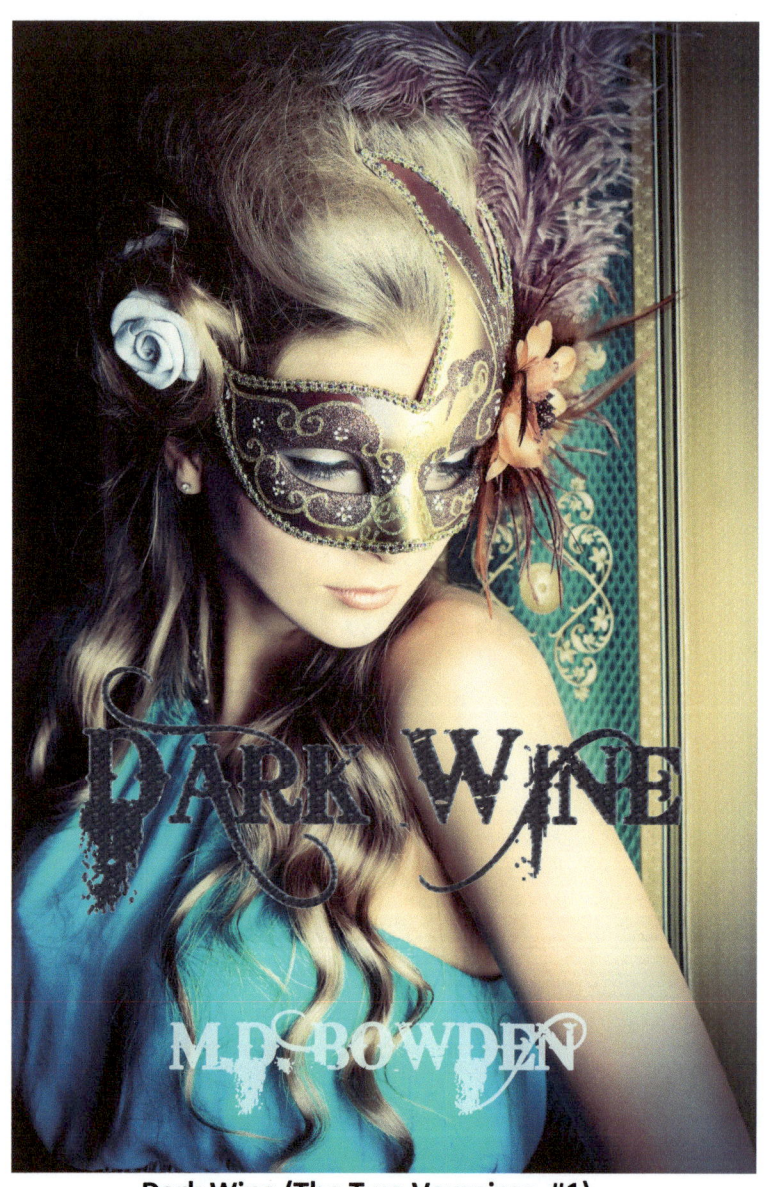

Dark Wine (The Two Vampires, #1)

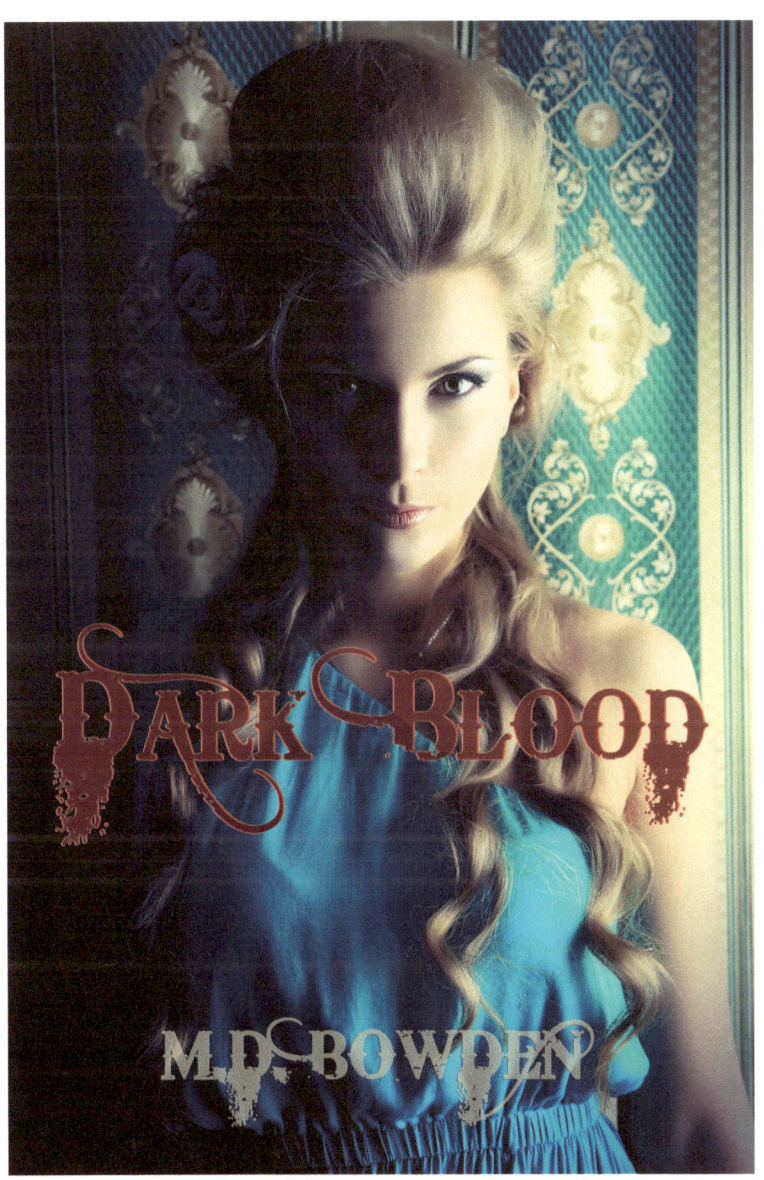

Dark Blood (The Two Vampires, #2)

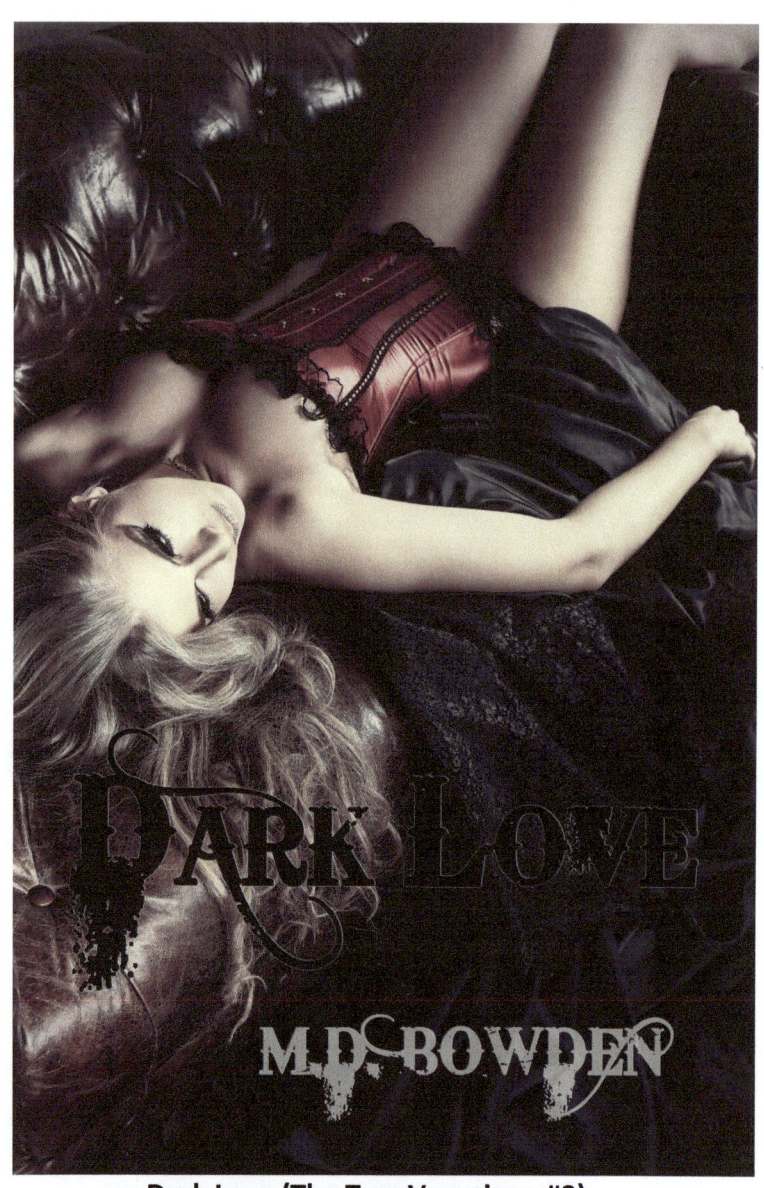

Dark Love (The Two Vampires, #3)

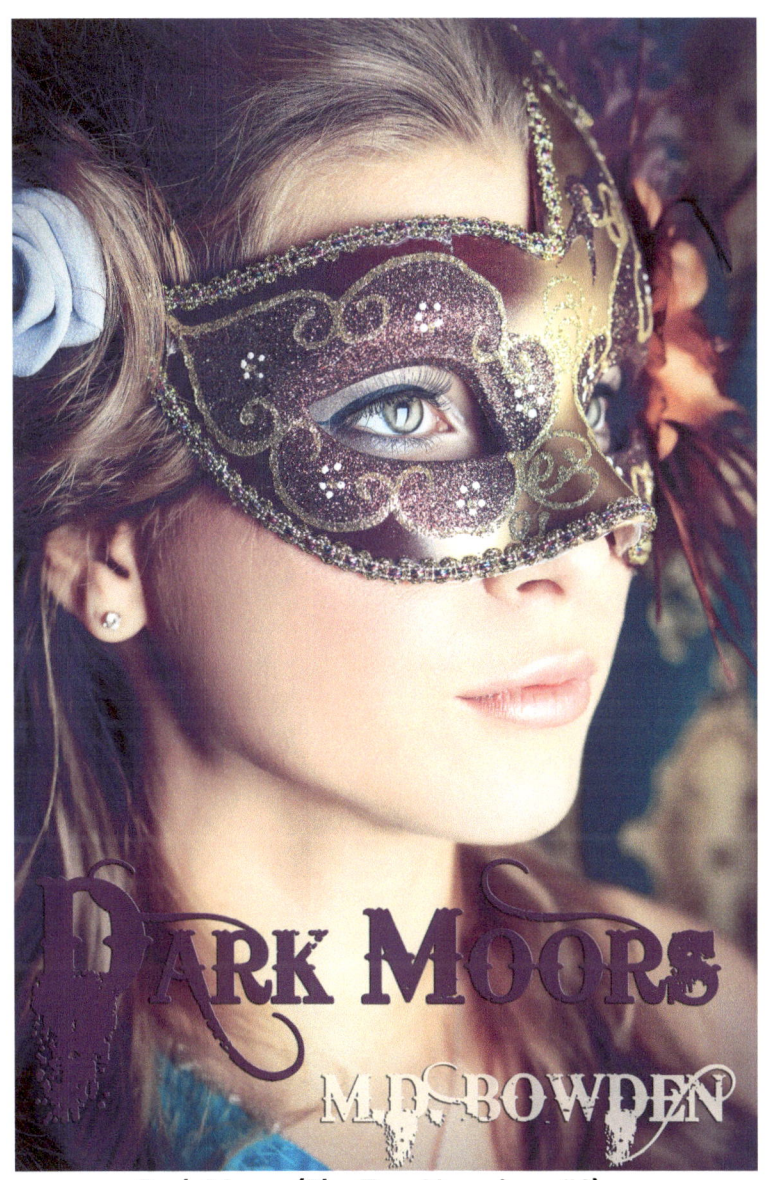

Dark Moors (The Two Vampires, #4)

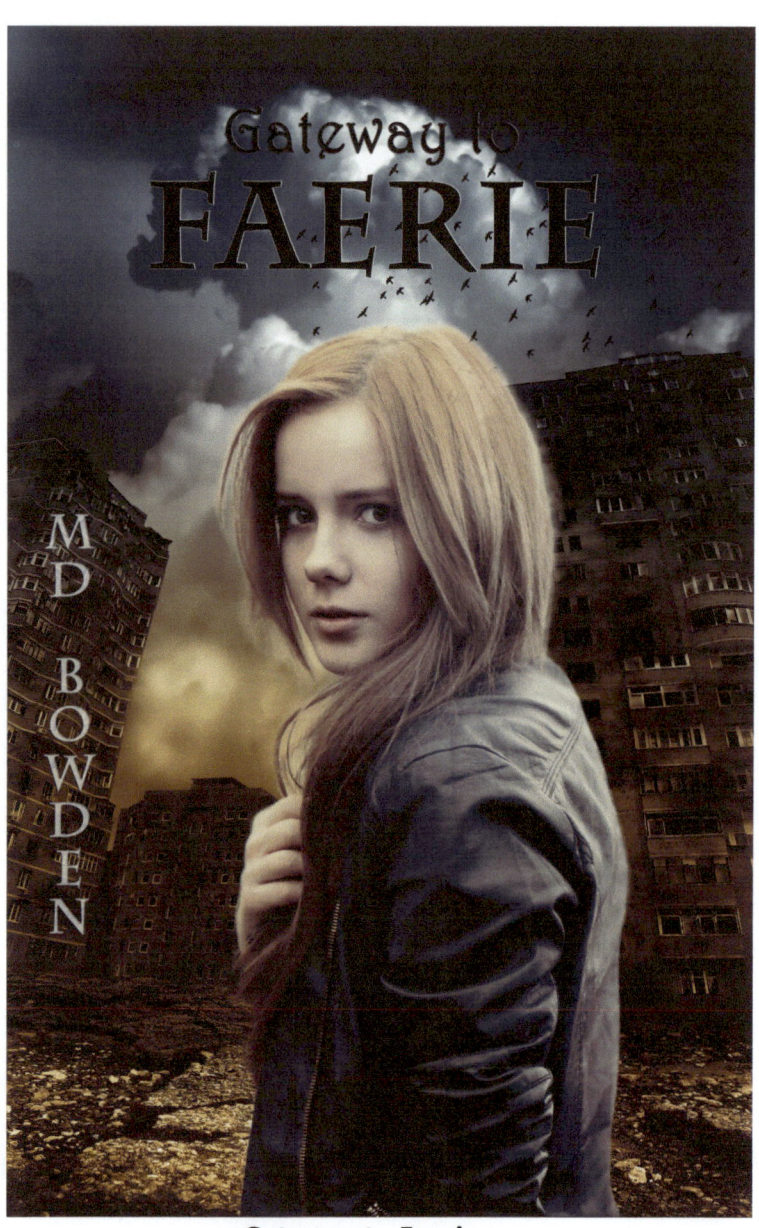

Gateway to Faerie

Read on for a taster from M.D. Bowden's new release:

Gateway to Faerie...

Chapter 1: Skries

I felt so alive this morning when I woke up, now I feel awful. My head is pounding and my muscles aching after a hard training session with my father.

He's at work now and I am left alone to study, but it's tricky with this stupid headache. I wish it would leave me alone so I could concentrate.

I stare down at my text book, not taking in the words in front of me. It's a history volume, exam's next week. I *really* must focus. I get the general topic, but it's the details I'm fuzzy on, the bits that matter when it comes to the test.

The ridiculous thing is, this is what I should be good at— my dad has explained it to me enough times. The thing is, I switch off as soon as he starts talking about history.

He is a history professor, well, more of a researcher really, although he does give the occasional lecture. It's probably that which puts me off, the serious tone he adopts as soon as he starts talking about *his* favourite subject, the faraway look in his eye.

He says that this stuff I'm learning is a load of crap anyway, that the real reason the planet is now so empty, so lacking in crowds and communities, is far darker.

Far scarier.

It's not in the history books because if people knew the truth they wouldn't be able to go about their day to day lives, they would just be too freaked out, and what is left of society would crumble.

That stuff is easier to remember, because it's real. Learning history that I know is fake does not come naturally to me.

I shift my bum, trying to get more comfortable on the granite rock I'm perched on, and stretch my back, before refocusing on the book on my lap.

The book is made of bleached white paper which is still crisp and smells fresh. It's one of the newest ones I own.

My father says it's important that I learn this stuff so I can get a decent job, like him, and that I never tell anybody what he's told me.

I don't know what would happen if I did.

What I do know though, is that if I don't pass my exams, if I can't get a job, the government won't help me. I will have to look after myself.

That's why I'm out here sitting on this uncomfortable stone. I am hoping some kind of animal will approach the bait; freshly cut carrot I grew in our garden. I've laid it out in a secluded corner that's protected by rocks and ferns, and in my direct line of sight.

I'm hoping to catch a rabbit, as they're my favourite. Then I can kill it and we will have meat for dinner.

My dad has taught me well, and I hunt frequently, so at least if I don't get a job I will be able to survive, I will be able to eat, and stand up for myself in a fight.

Unfortunately nothing is approaching the bait yet, so I return my attention to my book, rubbing my temples as I do.

I force myself to read the words on the open page . . .

~

'In the year 2046 the government of England refused to play a part in the war that was rapidly consuming the European nations, having spread from the Middle East. The leading party, Labour, thought that if it abstained from action it would not be a target.

The war spread quicker than anyone could have imagined, governments losing control as chemical agents started to be employed as the weapon of choice by multiple countries.

Nobody knew who was in control anymore, or who the enemy was.

Paranoia spread, and it wasn't long before France started to suspect that England was collecting their own supply of noxious nerve agents, and grew fearful that they would be the target, as France had recently destroyed the cities of Spain and Germany with nuclear weapons.'

~

I glance up at the bait, and around at my surroundings—water trickling around mossy boulders and flowing softly over the stream-bed, and the lush summer leaves overhead, gently moving in the wind.

Any excuse for a break.

No sign of life yet so I refocus on the book in front of me.

~

'England had not been accumulating weapons, but that did not stop France.

In 2046 France fought Scandinavia, defending itself against the repeated attacks it had suffered. After months of small invasions, they had still not won, so once again they deployed more nuclear weapons.

After France had taken down the countries surrounding it on land, it turned its full attention to England and targeted London with a powerful nuclear bomb.

Survivors from neighbouring counties fled, but many were suffering the effects of radiation sickness, and millions of people died. Those who didn't die fought each other for food, and anarchy spread through the country.

No-more attacks came from the government in France, who were themselves destroyed in an attack originating in Asia.

However, the damage was already done. The majority of the English governing party had been killed, and imports had stopped due to the fighting that was still rife in China and America.

Countless people died in a struggle to gather food as a famine took hold, and many died of starvation.'

~

I squeeze my eyes shut and rub my temples again, and look back towards the slices of carrot. I stare at them, only half seeing what's before me, as I think about what I've read, and why I find it so hard to remember it all.

It's the dates, I think. Dates that are so long ago, and countries I've never been to.

I've never been anywhere beyond where I travel on my own two feet, and occasional trips by train to the city of Exeter, where my father works, where he is now. It's one of the few remaining cities in England.

That's as far as I've ever been, and it only took about twenty minutes to get there.

No-one goes abroad anymore, how would they? More to the point—why would they? Europe is in ruins. There are no-longer beautiful cities with outstanding architecture. They are all gone, ransacked and deserted.

Of course, some people do still live there, but they are said to be savage and murderous.

No-one could afford to go further afield, and anyway, no-one even knows much about America or any other continents these days. I certainly don't. I read somewhere that a long time ago people used to travel to other countries all the time, but that world has ceased to exist.

Everybody still feels the after effects of the war, still lives in the world that was left behind. It just wasn't the war in my book. Far from it.

It was the war against Faerie.

The faeries that came from another world, another dimension.

Dad says that there is some truth in the made up history, in the sequence of events, the countries that fell first. Only they didn't fall to nuclear war, they fell as faerie after faerie came through the gate that had opened to their dimension, like a portal that had got jammed wide-open, and no-body could shut it.

The world was overcome, one country at a time, as these faerie's trashed houses and killed the people within. They torched cities, possessed people, controlled them, exchanged babies for changelings, and made people do bad things.

Dad says that these things did happen on the dates in my book, but they are still meaningless to me—this all happened over two hundred years ago! And anyway, what does it matter if I remember some stupid dates or not, or know which countries fell first? It won't make things any better now.

Dad says that the gate got closed in the end, somehow. That's what he's researching, well, one of the things. He found some ancient papers at the university that describe the faerie invasion, and dad is trying to find out how it ended, in case it ever happens again.

He thinks we need to be prepared.

That's why he trains me so hard, why he's always pushing me to do better. If it happens again he doesn't want me to suffer the same death that millions before me succumbed to. He wants me to live.

In fact, he's been talking about it more and more recently, pushing me harder than ever. It's almost as though he believes something bad is going to happen soon.

My eyes snap into focus as the ferns, near the bait I set, move apart. A soft grey rabbit pushes his nose through and approaches the carrots.

I stay stock still as he looks up to check that it is safe, before lowering his mouth and starting to nibble on the food.

I slowly slide the gun out of its belt and point it at the chewing ball of cuteness, then fire. A net launches from the barrel and wraps itself around the creature.

I jump to my feet, letting the gun fall to the ground, and pounce on the wriggling rabbit before it breaks free. I draw back a corner of the net and, taking a deep breath, stick a hand in fast, getting a firm hold around its belly to stop it squirming free.

Its fur is soft beneath my hands. I feel a moment of regret and I hesitate, inadvertently allowing the rabbit another attempt to escape. I grip it tightly again, take a short pause, take another deep breath, quickly reach for its neck, and snap.

I cringe.

I hate doing that, but I know I have to if I'm going to have meat for dinner.

I pick up the net and fold it carefully into the correct position for using again, then get down onto my knees next to the gun and insert the net back into the barrel. I slip the gun into my belt for safekeeping.

I wipe the thin layer of perspiration from my forehead and take yet another deep breath to steady myself. I did it. My father and I will have rabbit for dinner.

It would be even better if we had two.

I decide to leave the carrot in place, and try for a second bunny, but first I need to put the dead one somewhere cool so it doesn't go off in the heat.

I rustle in my pack for my cool bag, finding it folded at the bottom beneath my other book and supplies. I pull it out and shake it open, before gently placing the body of the rabbit inside.

I pick up my history book and slide it into my pack, along-side a maths one, and squeeze the cool bag back in too, before strapping the bag closed and shrugging it onto my back.

I glance down at the carrot, hoping I don't miss an opportunity to catch one while I'm gone, then I head off further from home.

I'm walking in the direction of a cave where I have set an old metal box for the express purpose of storing any animals I catch. It's not far away, ten minutes down-stream, set back in an enormous rock, and surrounded by boulders, trees and ferns.

The path stays close to the stream as I go. It is rocky so I keep glancing down to make sure I don't trip.

As I walk I think back to my earlier training.

My dad shakes me awake, "Fayth—time for action!" he compels me.

Ugh, how does he have this much enthusiasm, so early in the morning?

As my senses kick in I smell potatoes frying on the stove, and my stomach grumbles. This is enough to make me open my eyes, just as my father starts to shake my arm a second time.

I see his face before mine, in shadow in the early morning light, his mouth crinkling into a genuine smile, and deep chocolate coloured eyes radiating warmth.

He leaves the room and I hear him return to his cooking, as I push myself to my elbows and stifle a yawn.

This happens every other weekday. My dad wakes me ridiculously early so we can eat breakfast together, and then train, all before he leaves for work and I set out for school.

That was until recently anyway. As I'm approaching my final exams, and I don't have to go to any-more classes, I am left to revise at home.

After the exams I won't have to ever return to the school again. I grin. The joy this brings me releases a surge of energy, enough to finally motivate me to clamber from beneath the covers, quickly wash and dress, then jog down the stairs—reaching the kitchen just as my father is placing my eggs and potatoes on a plate.

There is already a glass of cool milk beside it, so I give my father a one armed hug as he dishes up his own food, before sliding onto a stool and tucking into mine.

It is warm and deliciously fresh, the eggs are from our own chickens, the potatoes dug up yesterday from the garden.

We exchanged surplus eggs for milk with Ewan Ford, a friend of dad's. The only thing we had to buy for this meal was the cooking oil.

As I finish my food I look up to my dad. He hasn't even sat down, but is leaning back against the counter, tucking in as he stands, watching me with a thoughtful frown.

"What is it?" I ask.

He swallows his food and takes a drink of milk before answering. "Just thinking about your future—what you are going to do after your exams . . ."

My feelings darken. It's all very well being happy I will no-longer have to go to school, with its practically totalitarian regime of work, silence and punishment, but that doesn't mean that whatever I do next will be any easier. That I will even find *anything* to do.

I shrug, assuming he's not expecting an answer, and glug back the last of my milk.

"What shall we start with this morning?" I ask, deflecting his thoughts.

He looks away, out of the window to the street, and watches as a neighbour empties vegetable cuttings onto a compost heap, to the side of her house.

"Let's go to the bottom of the garden and practice shooting, then we can do circuits," he finally responds.

I wonder at his mood, he seems troubled, but maybe he's still thinking of my future, so I decide not to broach the subject.

I simply say, "OK," and rise from my stool to show I am ready.

It's not long until I'm standing next to my father, a shot gun held firmly in my grip as I focus on a target he has set.

He is always challenging me, setting targets that are smaller or further away. He's even set up a rope, dangling from a high branch off one of our trees, to swing targets off. That is the hardest challenge I face. But today he's chosen precision as my skill to develop and I am focusing on an old ball that he has balanced on a post.

I am far enough away from it that I have to use every ounce of concentration I possess.

When I am ready, I squeeze the trigger. The force of the bullet leaving the gun makes my arms shake.

I rub my wrist with my free hand and look to the target. It is still there.

I missed.

I return to the present when I recognise I am close to the cave.

I turn from my path and follow a thin stream, stepping in the shallow water as there is no-where else to tread, and ducking so as not to hit my head on the tree branches that obscure the cave from sight when on the main path.

I originally found the cave in winter, when the trees had shed their leaves, removing their protective embrace.

I look up as the barely there stream turns into a trickle, falling over the mouth of the cave.

I sidestep the water and duck into the cool darkness beyond, fumbling at the catch to the metal box. When it is open I retrieve the rabbit from my pack and place it inside, where it will be safe until I come back for it later, when the day has started to lose its heat.

I trace my footsteps back to my seat near the carrot. I sigh, relieved. It looks like it has gone untouched.

The rock I am sat on is under the shelter of a tree, providing some relief from the warmth of the day. I am wearing black trousers, which don't help keep me cool in the sun, probably a mistake, but I like the protection these ones bring—they are durable and prevent me getting scratched by brambles in the woods, or thistles on the moor. They also have plenty of pockets, useful for storing bits of my survival gear, and fit well with the belt which holds my weapons.

I pull out my history book and force my eyes back to the page once again. I scan the lines, seeing the words, but not absorbing their meaning.

I hear a rustle in the trees and glance back towards its source, but can't get sight of what caused it. It was probably a deer, or maybe just a large bird. I crane my neck around, trying to verify my suspicions, but am unsuccessful.

I look back at my book but feel a prickle of unease as I do, and glance around again. I shake the feeling away, not wanting to be paranoid, and focus back on my work.

When the light starts to dim under the trees, I know it's time to stop what I'm doing, and give up hope of catching a second rabbit. I scoop up the left-over carrot as I don't want to waste it—I can feed some to our pig at home—and take a sip of water from my bottle, before making sure everything I brought is back in my bag and on my back.

I return to the cave and retrieve the rabbit from the metal box, and add that to my possessions in my pack, before starting my trek back towards Okehaven, and my home.

I follow the stream uphill until I'm out of the trees, and prickly gorse borders the path instead. It becomes steep and I take care as I clamber up rocks, until the path becomes level again.

I look out across the valley ahead as the sun starts to set, and the sky is streaked with red. I speed up, eager to reach the main path—the old road—before night sets in.

The old road is still some way ahead.

As I start to descend into the valley I hear a scuffling in the bushes. I can't help but glance nervously over my shoulder.

Trees cast shadows behind me and, even if there is someone there, it would be easy for them to blend into the landscape, for me not to notice.

I keep going, starting to feel weary, and hungry, and I try to ignore my fears. I am used to walking by myself at night, but that doesn't mean it doesn't bother me. It's not hard for some small thing to trigger my imagination to go into overdrive, and then the fear starts to escalate.

I take a deep breath, determined that won't happen this time.

When I reach the place to cross the stream I eye up the bridge. It almost looks safe, but the wood is crumbling so I decide not to risk it.

Instead I tread carefully through the water, making sure I step in the shallowest places so it doesn't go over the top of my boots. They are leather, but treated well, so pretty good at repelling water.

I reach the other side and place my hands on my knees as I climb another steep hill. I'm struggling for breath as I reach the top and stop for a break, looking back behind me as the sun finally disappears over the moorland horizon.

Nothing else has given me cause for concern and, despite the approaching darkness; I am feeling a little more confident. As I set foot on the old road I start gently jogging to get home faster.

My dad will be back soon, returning from Exeter by train, and he will be hungry too as today he had to work late.

My thoughts turn to preparing the rabbit and making a stew, and my stomach rumbles with hunger.

As darkness surrounds me I start to ascend the final hill before home. My father and I live right on the edge of town. Where we live it almost feels like a hamlet, or small village, as the houses are widely spread and everyone has large gardens.

Further into the centre of Okehaven the houses are more tightly packed, and people struggle to grow enough food to supplement what they can afford to buy.

The train station is in the centre so I won't cross paths with my dad until we meet at our cosy house. I can't wait to get there now, to take off my pack and stretch my shoulders, but I am getting tired so I slow my pace, and once again recover my breath.

As I round the final corner, before I will see my home, something grabs me from behind. I instantly panic. An arm firmly wraps around both of mine, pinning them to my side, at the same time as fingers cover my mouth so I can't shout out.

I struggle silently, trying to get my arms free, but my breath halts in my chest when I see a shadow cross the dimly lit path about a hundred metres ahead.

I freeze, but although I've stopped struggling, I am not let free.

I see another shadow materialise from behind a tree, and yet another come out from behind our neighbour's house.

I strain my eyes to see clearly, my heart pounding in my chest, not knowing if I'm in danger from the shadows, or from the person restraining me.

At least whoever is holding me doesn't seem bent on causing pain, so I decide to hope they are trying to keep me safe.

Then I spot my father's head as he rounds the hill, and his body comes into sight as he nears our front path.

I start to struggle again, but am held even tighter.

Dad looks content, unaware of the danger. I want to get to him, to whisk him inside and away from the shadows.

I try to shout through the fingers that are over my mouth, to warn him, but before a sound starts to rise in my throat, a fierce whisper stops me.

"They're after you, stay quiet."

No sound leaves my lips, but as the first shadow approaches my father, I can just see his face turn to fear. Some kind of exchange occurs, but I can't hear what is said.

I see my father step back, but another shadow is behind him.

I resume my struggles, trying to move forward, to help, but another whisper cuts me off.

"They are too dangerous, you can't do anything to help," and then a gentler whisper of, "I'm sorry," as the shadow behind my father steps up to him and draws a blade across his throat.

My eyes widen as blood spills and my father crumples to his knees, then falls flat on his face. I hear a crunch as his glasses break, and shock pervades my system.

I am still, my throat feels cut too, I can't think, function.

I see the shadows, wraiths, return to the corners and nooks surrounding my house, as whoever is holding me pulls me further away, until I can no longer see my house, can no longer see my fallen father.

End of Sample
Gateway to Faerie is available to purchase from all main
ebook retailers

AUTHOR BIO

M.D. BOWDEN lives in England with her partner and two young children. She enjoys spending time with her family, in the sea, on the cliffs, and reading as much fantasy as she can get her hands on.

Twitter: https://twitter.com/manderbowden81

Facebook: http://www.facebook.com/mdBowden81

Smashwords:
https://www.smashwords.com/profile/view/mdBOWDEN

www.ingramcontent.com/pod-product-compliance
Lightning Source LLC
Chambersburg PA
CBHW040321010626
45792CB00024B/2080